Autoimmune Disease Inflammation Diet

Natural Pain Relief and Disease Control

By Mary Solomon

2nd Edition

Contents

Introduction

Over time, it has become clearer to see that many serious illnesses have one thing as their root cause – chronic inflammation. Even diseases such as Alzheimer's, heart disease and a large number of cancers can be blamed, at least in part on inflammation. But, do you really know what this inflammation is? Sure, you've seen it on your skin – red, swollen, painful and hot patches but did you know that the same thing happens inside your body as well?

Inflammation is vital to the body, it is required for healing it brings a certain amount of nourishment and immune system activity to an area of the body that has been injured or is the site of an infection. But, we only need a certain amount. When we get too much inflammation in our bodies or it is serving no real purpose, then it becomes a problem; then it starts to damage our bodies form the inside out, damage that can't see, illnesses that just put down to bad luck or fate.

This inflammation is caused by a lot of different things – stress, anxiety, lack of exercise, genetic predisposition and exposure to toxins like tobacco smoke. Your diet also plays a very big role and it is vital that you learn exactly how specific foods affect and influence inflammation in the body if you want to learn how to control it.

That's why you need to know about the anti-inflammatory diet – not a diet, as you would automatically think, although it is possible to lose weight if you follow it. It also isn't a fad diet that you stay on for a couple of weeks. Instead, it is a lifestyle, a lifelong one in which you learn how to choose and prepare foods based on how they help your body. As well as helping to influence levels of inflammation in the body, this diet will also give you access to a steady stream of energy and the right levels of nutrients, minerals, vitamins, fiber, phytonutrients and essential fatty acids – all the things needed to stay healthy.

Chapter 1: Autoimmune Diseases and Inflammation

The human immune system is a collection of certain chemicals and cells that fight and protect our bodies against the infections that cause bacteria and viruses. As such, the immune system plays a vital role in protecting us against microbial infections. In autoimmune disorders, the immune system fails to function properly and it mistakenly takes the body's own cells and tissues as foreign invaders and starts killing them. What happens when the immune system fails to differentiate between its own cells and foreign invaders? When this happens, the affected body forms autoantibodies that mistakenly attack the body's own cells. On the other side, the regulatory T cells fail to do their job in keeping the immune system in line. This results in a mistaken attack on your body's own cells.

The damage that results from this process is known as an autoimmune disease. Autoimmune disorders are mainly divided into 2 categories: Organ specific autoimmune disorders, in which mainly one organ is affected by the disorder, the other is non-organ specific autoimmune disorder that can affect multiple organs and systems. There are about 80 autoimmune disorders, which can range from minor to disabling in severity, based on the type of affected organ and the degree of disability. Due to some unknown reasons, women are more likely to get autoimmune disorders than men, especially during childbearing periods; it is assumed the sex hormones might be one reason amongst the others. To date, there is no cure for autoimmune disorders, but with some treatment options, the symptoms of autoimmune disorders can be managed.

Autoimmune diseases are very common, affecting more than 23.5 million people in the USA alone. Autoimmune disorders are one of the leading causes of disability and death. As we all know, there are many (about 80) autoimmune disorders and some are very common, yet some autoimmune disorders are rare.

How Autoimmune Diseases Cause Inflammation

When an autoimmune disease occurs, it causes overproduction of chemokines and cytokines that leads to the inflammation of the body tissues. For instance, excess of cytokines in the joints can cause rheumatoid arthritis. This condition gets worse when chemokines bring more destructive components of the immune system, like T cells, macrophages and neutrophils, to the affected joints, intensifying the inflammatory response.

Who is at Risk of Getting Autoimmune Diseases?

Anyone can get autoimmune disorders, but certain people are at more risk.

1- Childbearing Women

Overall, due to some unknown reasons, more women (of childbearing age) than men get autoimmune diseases.

2- People Having a Positive Family History for Autoimmune Diseases

There are some autoimmune diseases that run in families, like multiple sclerosis and lupus. It is a common trend that some autoimmune diseases affect different members of a family. If a person inherits some genes from the family, that person has more chances of developing an autoimmune disease. However, a combination of genes and other factors can increase the chances of developing an autoimmune disease.

3- Environmental Triggers

Exposure to certain environmental triggers and exposures can lead to or worsen autoimmune disorders. Sunlight, certain solvents, bacterial and viral infections are associated with the development of some autoimmune diseases.

4- People of Certain Races

Some autoimmune diseases affect certain races more

severely than the others. For instance, lupus is more common and severe in Hispanic people and American African, and, similarly, type 1 Diabetes is more prevalent in white people compared to others.

Chapter 2: Diagnosis of Autoimmune Disorders

Generally, it is very hard to diagnose an autoimmune disease, especially when it is in its initial stages. Autoimmune diseases involving many organs and systems are very difficult to diagnose. Based on the type of autoimmune disorders, the diagnostic methods can involve:

- ❖ X-rays
- ❖ Biopsy
- ❖ Certain blood tests including those that can detect autoantibodies
- ❖ Physical examination
- ❖ Patient history
- ❖ Antinuclear Antibody Test
- ❖ Protein Electrophoresis
- ❖ Complement Test
- ❖ C Reactive Protein Test

Common Autoimmune Inflammatory Diseases

Autoimmune Hepatitis

Autoimmune hepatitis is a long lasting and chronic disorder in which the body's immune cells mistakenly attack the normal liver cells and components and cause liver damage and inflammation. Autoimmune hepatitis is a critical disorder that may become worse and severe over time if left untreated. If this condition gets prolonged, it may result in liver failure or cirrhosis. When scar tissue replaces normal liver cells and tissue, it blocks the normal blood flow through the liver and in this way, cirrhosis occurs. When liver fails to work optimally, it leads to the liver failure.

Common Causes of Autoimmune Hepatitis

Environmental triggers, genetic predisposition, autoimmunity or a combination of any of these factors may lead to autoimmune hepatitis.

Who is at More Risk of Getting this Autoimmune Disorder?

This chronic disorder can affect anybody at any age and in any ethnic group. But this disorder occurs mostly in females.

Types of Autoimmune Hepatitis

There are many types of autoimmune hepatitis. Type 1 autoimmune hepatitis can occur at any time and at any age, but it is more common in North America and most commonly affects adolescent and younger people. About 70% of people affected by this autoimmune disorder are females.

People suffering from autoimmune hepatitis commonly have some other autoimmune disease like:

- Graves' disease,
- Crohn's disease,
- Celiac disease,
- Proliferative glomerulonephritis,
- Sjogren's syndrome,
- Rheumatoid arthritis,
- Ulcerative colitis,
- Systemic lupus,
- Type one diabetes, etc.

Type 2 autoimmune hepatitis is not as common as type 1 and it mostly occurs in children. People having type 2 autoimmune hepatitis can have any of the above disorders.

Symptoms of autoimmune Hepatitis

- Jaundice or yellowish skin
- Dark urine and light colored stools
- Joint pain
- Fatigue
- Nausea
- Liver pain
- Less appetite or complete loss of appetite
- Skin rashes

Symptoms of autoimmune hepatitis can be very mild or severe. Some people may experience a mild flu, while others may not have any apparent symptom of this disorder when a healthcare professional diagnoses the disease. However, symptoms of the disease can develop later on.

Diagnosis of autoimmune Hepatitis

A health professional can make a diagnosis of the disease based on physical examination of the patient, patient's history, and blood examinations and via a liver biopsy.

Treatment of autoimmune Hepatitis

People having autoimmune hepatitis with few to mild symptoms may or may not need medical treatment. A health care provider can better decide about the treatment based on medical examinations and patient's history. In people suffering from the disease and having mild symptoms, this disorder might go into remission. Remission is a smaller period when the person may go symptom free and an improvement in liver function is noted in his blood test and liver biopsy.

Corticosteroids

Corticosteroids are drugs that reduce the swelling and suppress the activity of the immune system. Health care professionals prescribe corticosteroids (usually prednisone) for the treatment of both types of autoimmune hepatitis. Initially, a high dose is given to patients, which is decreased as symptoms are controlled.

Immunosuppressants

Drugs that suppress the activity of the immune system prevent the immune system from making autoantibodies and block the autoimmune response that leads to the inflammation. Azathioprine is the drug in this class mostly used by the health professionals, along with prednisone to treat this deadly disorder.

There are some mild to severe side effects associated with the use of these drugs, therefore health care professionals monitor the patients closely and adjust the dose accordingly.

Liver Transplant

When autoimmune hepatitis reaches end stage liver failure or cirrhosis, a liver transplant becomes mandatory. It is a very complicated and expensive treatment approach. Liver transplant surgery is usually successful and the patient is advised to take prescription medicines for a long period to prevent transplant rejections and other infections.

Complications of autoimmune Hepatitis

People having autoimmune hepatitis are at a greater risk of getting liver cancer. A health professional continuously keeps on monitoring the patient with a liver ultrasound. Specialized and trained technicians or doctors do the ultrasound examination. The images obtained via ultrasound of the liver can tell about liver cancer or the presence of cancerous tissues in the liver.

Rheumatoid Arthritis

Rheumatoid arthritis is an autoimmune, chronic, long lasting, disabling, progressive and inflammatory disease that is known to cause pain in the joints and inflammation in the tissues that surround the joints; this disease may also affect some other body organs. This disease generally affects joints in the hands and feet, but it may affect any joints in the human body. Stiff joints, tiredness and feelings of being unwell are the most common problems that rheumatoid patients complaint.

People that suffer from this autoimmune disorder produce autoantibodies in their blood that misread their own body tissues as foreign invaders, attack and kill them, resulting in an inflammation. The immune system of rheumatoid patients affects the lining of the joints and causes them to become inflamed. Rheumatoid arthritis does not cause wear and tear damage like osteoarthritis, instead it attacks and destroys the lining of the joints that results in a painful swelling that can cause bone deformity and bone erosion. If left untreated, rheumatoid arthritis can cause permanent joints damage.

Rheumatoid arthritis is a systemic illness. It affects joints and the entire body as well. Rheumatoid arthritis can affect multiple organs in the body. The patients sometimes may experience fever and fatigue. Rheumatoid arthritis patients are at a greater risk of getting a heart attack compared to other people.

According to John Hopkins Arthritis Center, USA
   ❖ Approximately 1-2% people of the world are affected by rheumatoid arthritis
   ❖ Prevalence of rheumatoid arthritis increases with age, about 5% women over 55 years are affected by this disorder
   ❖ In the United Sates, about 70 people are affected in every 100,000 people.

- ❖ Smokers are more likely to get rheumatoid arthritis (4 times higher chances) than non-smokers
- ❖ Rheumatoid arthritis is more common than multiple sclerosis and leukemia. But unfortunately, the severity of its effects and awareness is more restricted to the patients, their relatives and caregivers as the public is not well aware of this disabling disorder.
- ❖ Symptoms of the disease will not always stay active as they go and come. At some point, the symptoms might be mild, but sometimes they may be very painful and severe. A patient may have a sudden outbreak of the disease
- ❖ Although there is no known cure for this disease, a proper diagnosis and treatment may slow down the progression of the disease and make the symptoms less severe and easier to live with.

Signs and Symptoms

We hear and read these words repeatedly. What is the difference between a sign and a symptom? Well, it is pretty simple. A symptom is what a patient feels and experiences and a sign is what other people can see like a doctor. For example, in rheumatoid arthritis, we can say joint pain is a symptom and an inflammation is a sign.

As we all know, rheumatoid arthritis is a chronic and long lasting disease. Different people may experience this disorder differently and might experience different symptoms. In some patients, symptoms may come and go, while others may experience its symptoms continuously. A patient who experiences a sudden severe onset of this disorder may go to sleep healthy but may get up the next morning having severe rheumatoid pain and may also not be able to get out of the bed.

In most cases, rheumatoid arthritis begins quietly. Signs and symptoms of the disease develop gradually over a period of weeks or months. Initially, the patient might experience pain and stiffness in one joint that is usually associated with severe pain when the patient tries to move that joint. Rheumatoid pain is usually felt in small joints at the beginning like joints in the toes and fingers. Numbers of affected joints are not the same in all cases, but it affects at least five joints simultaneously. Rheumatoid arthritis is a polyarthritis disease, which means it affects more and more joints with the passage of time.

Commonly Affected Joints
- Basic and middle joints of the finger
- Ankles
- Knees
- Elbow
- Shoulders
- Non-Specific Symptoms that might appear months before the other symptoms
- Low grade fever
- Depression

- Fatigue
- Malaise

Remission of Symptoms

Symptoms of this auto inflammatory disease are not steady as they come and go at times. There might be few symptoms for months for the patient and after that period, the patient might experience a sudden outbreak of the symptoms.

Other Systems/Organs of the Body that can be affected

As we know, rheumatoid arthritis is a systemic illness, so it can affect multiple organs of the body.

Inflammation in the Cricoarytenoid Joint

Cricoarytenoid joint is present in the larynx. When inflammation occurs in this joint, it may cause hoarseness.

Nodular Lesions

About 25% of rheumatoid patients develop lumps under the skin. These lumps usually appear on the skin over the forearms and elbows. They are rarely painful and usually colorless in appearance.

Risk Factors

What is a risk factor for any disease? Well, a risk factor could be anything that increases the likelihood of getting any disease or condition. For example, cigarette smoking increases the risk of developing lung cancer and obesity is associated with increased risk of type 2 diabetes.

The following are the risk factors for rheumatoid arthritis:

Hormones

Certain hormones play a role in the development of rheumatoid arthritis. A low testosterone level in males is a sign of getting rheumatoid arthritis in the future.

Age

Although any person of any age can develop this disease, people aged between 40-60 are at more risk than the others.

Genetics

Although rheumatoid arthritis is not a hereditary disease, some people have a genetic predisposition to develop this disorder. People having a close family member with rheumatoid arthritis are at a greater risk of developing this disorder.

Gender

According to the Mayo Clinic, rheumatoid arthritis affects women two to three times more than men. This might be because of the hormone estrogen, however, this is still needs to be proved as it is still a theory.

Smoking

Smoking is associated with increased risk of developing rheumatoid arthritis, so smokers have a higher risk for rheumatoid arthritis.

Causes

Rheumatoid arthritis occurs when the immune system mistakenly starts attacking the lining of the membranes that surrounds the joints (also known as synovium). As a result of this destruction of the synovium, the inflammation makes the synovium thicker and can ultimately destroy the bone and cartilage within the joints. Ligaments and tendons become weak and stretch, and in this way, the joint deforms and loses its alignment and shape. Still nobody knows what starts this process, but it is believed that genetics might play a role here. Although inherited genes do not cause rheumatoid arthritis, yet they can make a person more susceptible to developing this disease.

Complications of Rheumatoid Arthritis

- **Increased Risk for Lung Disease**

As rheumatoid arthritis is an inflammatory disease, people having this disease have an increased risk of developing inflammation and scarring of the lungs, which might lead to shortness of breath.

- **Osteoporosis**

Rheumatoid arthritis and medicines used for the treatment of this disease can increase the risk for developing osteoporosis.

- **Increased Risk of Heart Diseases**

Rheumatoid arthritis can harden and block the heart arteries. It can also increase the risk of inflammation of the sac that encloses the heart.

- **Carpel Tunnel Syndrome**

Rheumatoid arthritis can increase the risk of developing carpel tunnel syndrome

Diagnosis of Rheumatoid Arthritis

During early phases, this disease is very difficult to diagnose. Its main signs and symptoms (stiffness and inflammation) are just like the signs and symptoms of many other conditions. A doctor will carry out a physical examination to see whether a patient is suffering from the disease or not. The doctor will examine the joints to see whether they are inflamed or not and see the movability of the joints. The patient will be asked about the symptoms. The patient should tell the doctor about all signs and symptoms for a correct diagnosis.

- Diagnostic Blood Tests
- ESR
    Blood test for anemia
- C reactive protein
- Rheumatoid factor test
- MRI
- X-rays and image scans

How to Confirm Rheumatoid Arthritis?

In 1987, the American College of Rheumatology defined the classification criteria for rheumatoid arthritis

- Possible joint erosion suggested by radiological findings
- Morning stiffness which lasts for more than an hour for a period of six weeks
- Arthritis and soft tissue swelling should be present in more than 3 of 14 joints/joints groups for a period of at least 6 weeks
- Rheumatoid factor should be greater than 95 percentile

- Subcutaneous nodules should be present in specific areas
- Symmetric arthritis should be present for a period of 6 weeks or more

To confirm the presence of rheumatoid arthritis, at least four above conditions should be met. Initially, these criteria were for research rather than for diagnostic purposes. Sometimes the condition might get worse if the doctor waits to meet all criteria set by American College of Rheumatology.

Distinguishing Rheumatoid Arthritis

There are some other conditions that may also cause joint pain:

- ❖ Gonococcal arthritis
- ❖ Sarcoidosis
- ❖ Whippele's disease
- ❖ Acute rheumatic fever

Treatment Approaches for Rheumatoid Arthritis

Unfortunately, to date, there is no cure available for rheumatoid arthritis. The treatment options aimed at reducing the inflammation, joints pain, slowing down the joints deformation or to limit any sort of disability because of rheumatoid arthritis. An occupational therapist and a physiotherapist can help the patients on how to protect their joints. Based on the time of diagnosis (meaning whether the disease was diagnosed at an early stage or not) and the degree of damage, surgery sometimes might be necessary.

Commonly used drugs

- Corticosteroids
- NSAIDS
- Disease Modifying anti rheumatic drugs
- Immunosuppressant's
- Occupational therapy
- Surgery
- Lifestyle modification (like acupuncture, massage, electrotherapy etc.)

Lupus

Lupus is an autoimmune inflammatory disease in which the body's immune system becomes overactive and mistakenly starts killing healthy and normal tissues. As a result of this, symptoms like swelling, inflammation and damage to the lungs, kidneys, heart, skin and joints start appearing in the affected individuals.

Different Types of Lupus

Although there are various types of lupus, the type we usually refer is SLE or systemic lupus erythematosus. Discoid lupus erythematosus, neonatal lupus and drug-induced lupus are among the other types.

Discoid Lupus Erythematosus

This type of lupus is limited to the skin. It is characterized by a rash that can appear on the scalp, face and neck, yet it does not affect the internal organs. Normally, no more than 10% people who get this go on to get systemic lupus erythematosus. However, there is no way to predict or stop the progression of the disease.

Drug Induced Erythematosus

This type of lupus occurs because of the reaction with some prescription drugs and its symptoms are similar to systemic lupus erythematosus. This type of lupus is associated with hydralazine and procainamide use, but there are nearly 400 other medications that might cause this form of lupus. This type of lupus subsides after patient stops taking the triggering medicines.

Neonatal Lupus

This rare type of lupus occurs when a mother passes autoantibodies to the fetus. The newborn or unborn fetus can get skin rashes along with some other blood and heart complications. The appeared rashes usually disappear or fade within the first six months of the child's life.

Systemic Erythematous Lupus

It is the more common and severe form of systemic lupus and it can affect any part or organ of the body. Having SLE, some people might only show inflammation and other symptoms in joints and skin, while others can have inflammation in joints, skin or any other organ of the body. This type of lupus is characterized by some flare up periods along with remission periods.

Who can get Lupus?

About 1.5 to 2 million US people suffer from any type of lupus according to the Lupus Foundation of America. Among Northern Europeans, some form of lupus affects 40 people out of every 100,000. In African- Americans, lupus affects 200 people out of 100,000. Although lupus can affect males and females, females have 9 times more chances of getting this autoimmune disease. High mortality rates and a more severe form of this disorder is usually diagnosed in African American women. It mainly affects people of 15-45 years of age. Some prescription medicines, exposure to sunlight and chemicals are among the other risk factors.

Causative Agents of the Disease

Like many other autoimmune diseases, the real cause of this disease is still unknown; however, many healthcare professionals believe that it occurs because of certain genetic and environmental factors. As lupus continues in families, many doctors believe that people inherit a genetic pre disposition to this disease from their families. It is believed that people who inherit genetic pre disposition to this disease develop it only when they are exposed to certain environmental triggers. The higher risk of lupus in females indicates that certain hormones might play a role in the development of this disease.

Some Triggering Environmental Factors

- Smoking
- Extreme stress
- Being exposed to UV light
- Some sulpha and penicillin group medications
- Having some viral infections like parvovirus, hepatitis C etc.
- Signs and Symptoms of lupus
- Achy, swelled and painful joints.
- High fever (more than 38C)
- Swelling in the feet and hands because of kidney problems
- Butterfly like rashes in near and on the nose and cheeks
- Shortness of breath and chest pain
- Anemia
- Alopecia
- Light sensitivity

- Weight gain or weight gain
- Dry eyes
- Memory loss, anxiety and depression

Complications of Lupus

As lupus is an auto inflammatory disease, inflammation caused by lupus can affect different areas of the body.

Heart

Lupus can cause inflammation of arteries, heart membrane and heart muscles. Because of this inflammation, the chances of heart attack and heart diseases may increase significantly.

Lungs

Lupus increases the chances of developing inflammation in the lining of the chest cavity. This resulting inflammation can make the breathing process more painful. People having lupus become more susceptible to pneumonia.

Kidneys

Lupus can seriously damage the kidneys. Among lupus patients, kidney failure is one of the major reasons of death. Chest pain, vomiting, nausea, generalized itching, and leg edema are among the obvious signs of kidney problems.

Blood and Blood Vessels

People having lupus are at increased risk of getting blood problems like anemia, blood clotting and increased bleeding problems. Blood vessels may become inflamed because of this disorder.

Brain and Central Nervous System

People having lupus might get brain and CNS problems. Symptoms may include behavioral changes, dizziness, light headaches, hallucinations, strokes or seizure. Some people with lupus experience memory loss and problems in expressing their thoughts to other people.

Diagnosis of Lupus

Generally, it is not easy to diagnose lupus as its symptoms overlap with many other diseases and conditions. There is no single test that can confirm whether you have lupus or not. Anyhow, if you have symptoms of lupus, tell your doctor or physician right away. Your doctor will find out if you are suffering from lupus.

Blood and Urine Tests

Your doctor will go for an antinuclear antibody test. This test helps to find out whether anybody's immune system is making autoantibodies for lupus or not. Surprisingly, most people's ANA test is usually positive. However, a positive ANA (antinuclear antibody) test does not confirm lupus. About 10% healthy women show a positive ANA test while they do not have lupus.

Medical History

Tell your doctor about your symptom and signs. By having your medical history, your doctor can decide whether you are suffering from lupus or not.

Complete Physical Exam

A complete physical exam can help a doctor to diagnose this disease

Family History of Lupus or other Autoimmune Diseases

If you have a positive family history for lupus or any other autoimmune disease, tell your doctor about it. This might be helpful for your doctor to make a better diagnosis.

Kidney or Skin Biopsy

A kidney or skin biopsy can be helpful in the diagnosis of this disorder.

Treatment of Lupus

There is no known cure for lupus. Therefore, the goal of

the treatment is always to decrease the inflammation, ease the symptoms, decrease risk of organ damage, reduce flares and to treat the symptoms when they appear.

Classes of drugs commonly used for the treatment of lupus

- Immunosuppressants
- NSAIDS
- Corticosteroids
- BLyS- Specific Inhibitors
- Antimalarial medications
- Anti-inflammatory diets

Chapter 3: What Is Inflammation?

Inflammation is a normal response of the immune system against infections and injuries and nobody can heal without it. However, prolonged, chronic and uncontrolled inflammation can be painful, dangerous and can seriously harm the body. It is believed that inflammation plays a role in cancer, obesity and certain heart diseases. Therefore, it is very important to counter the inflammation to save the body from further complications and damages.

Because of advancements in medical sciences, many anti-inflammatory drugs promise to relieve the pain and decrease the inflammation. In this way, these medicines can stop resulting in allergic reactions and may be helpful in preventing further complications because of the inflammation. But on the other side, long-term use of anti-inflammatory drugs like steroids and NSAIDS are associated with many unwanted side effects along with the weakening of the immune system.

Fortunately, Nature has provided so many natural anti-inflammatory foods that do not have any side effects and they taste great as well. Furthermore, these natural foods are packed with so many essential and valuable nutrients and minerals. Along with their ability to reduce inflammation, these foods provide us essential vitamins, nutrients and boost our immune system. Eating anti-inflammatory foods can help to fight against certain diseases that are caused or worsened by inflammation.

How To Tell If You Are Suffering From Chronic Inflammation?

One of the first indicators that you are suffering from an inflammatory condition is a raised level of C-Protein in your blood. This protein is produced by your body in response to inflammation. According to research, carried out over a three-year period, CRP is the strongest predictor of heart diseases, compared to around 11 other indicators, including LDL, or bad, cholesterol.

If you have a strong family history of inflammatory conditions or heart disease, you should speak to your doctor and ask for a CRP test, no matter what age you are.

Foods to Avoid

There are a number of foods that can trigger

inflammation in the body. The worst are wheat, milk, eggs, meat, yeast and soybeans. Meat is full of arachidonic acid, which promotes inflammation, with beef being the highest in content. In fact, beef has more than twice the amount of arachidonic acid that lamb, chicken or pork has, Dairy products and eggs also contain this acid but in lower amounts.

All the health advice about using vegetable oils and margarine instead of rich fatty butter has turned out to be wrong and has led to a huge increase in the levels of omega-6, thus profiting inflammation. Oils such as corn, sunflower, peanut, soy, safflower and cottonseed are extremely high in omega-6.

Instead eat poultry that is free range – grass fed poultry is higher in omega-3 fatty acids, which help to fight the inflammation. Unless it upsets your stomach, dairy is fine in small amounts but look for eggs that contain extra omega-3. Avoid processed foods, sugary drinks, anything with refined white four and fried foods, especially potatoes.

Helpful Food Swaps

Heart disease, skin irritation, diabetes, irritable bowel syndrome, even general aches and pains can be caused by excessive inflammation in the body. Stress, not enough exercise and genetics can also contribute to chronic inflammation, as can a bad diet, full of sugary, processed, fried and flour laden foods. Replace some of the worst culprits with anti-inflammatory alternatives and notice the difference in a short space of time. These eight food swaps can put out the fire of inflammation:

- **Swap Cereal for Walnuts and Berries**

Whole-grain cereals might seem like a healthy choice but they are very high in carbohydrate and can cause blood sugar spikes, which lead to inflammation. If you need to start the day with something that is sweet and crunchy, swap your cereal for a bowl of chopped walnuts and berries. Berries contain antioxidants and natural sugars while the walnuts are packed with anti-inflammatory healthy fats.

- **Kick out the Eggs and Eat Greek Yoghurt**

Eggs are not a bad choice provided they have extra omega-3 in them but that is only a small percentage of eggs sold. Instead, choose Greek yoghurt for your breakfast. It is lower in sugar than regular yoghurt, has double the amount of protein, and may help to cut down on insulin surges that can lead to inflammation. Add berries of your choice for a delicious breakfast or dessert.

- **Ditch the Sugar in Favor of Cinnamon**

Get rid of the refined white sugar you normally add to your coffee and try cinnamon instead. As well as being a sweet spice that adds plenty of flavor, it can also help to reduce inflammation. ¼ teaspoon per day is sufficient to get all the benefits.

- **Swap that Turkey Sandwich for a Bow of vegetarian Chili**

A lot of people eat protein of some description for lunch, whether it is meat, fish or chicken but, if you want to stay free of inflammation, choose a vegetable chili instead. Legumes are packed full of protein and eating them on a regular basis, with beans, can stop the sugar spikes that cause inflammation.

- **Olive Oil is Better Than a Creamy Salad Dressing**

Ok, so it might not sound as tasty, but store bought salad dressings are full of fat and sugar. Add a spoonful of extra virgin olive oil to your salad to stop inflammation from occurring. Spice it up with a bit of balsamic vinegar and fresh herbs.

- **Spread Avocado in Your Sandwich Instead of Mayonnaise**

Ditch the mayonnaise in your sandwich for a spoonful of avocado. It's just as creamy and it full of healthy fat and plenty of fiber – something mayonnaise doesn't have.

- **Use Spices Not Salt for Seasoning**

Too much salt can cause inflammation so cut back on the amount you eat and use spices like turmeric and chili powder, not to mention herbs to season your food.

Chapter 4: Changing Your Diet

With all this talk of inflammatory diets and how the food you eat could be doing you more harm than good, you might be wondering exactly what it is you can eat. The good news is, there is plenty of variety for you to choose from and including a good balance of them in your daily diet can help to reverse or prevent inflammation from occurring. Your diet is the safest way of treating inflammation as what you eat helps your body to make its own anti-inflammatory compounds. It is much easier to prepare your own meals at home, rather than eating out, when you first start to eat right to treat or prevent inflammation. That way, you get the ingredients right. The following is a helpful guide to the foods you should be eating if you suffer from high cholesterol, high triglycerides or C - reactive protein, all risk factors in inflammation:

- **Polyphenols.**

Polyphenols are anti-inflammatory Phytochemicals and you will find them in foods that are full of color, such as blackberries, blueberries, raspberries and strawberries. Berries also contain flavonoids that are called anthocyanin's that can help to protect against oxidative damage.

- **Quercetin.**

Quercitin is an anti-inflammatory compound as well as being a natural inhibitor for histamine. It is also one of the single most powerful flavonoids that you will find and it can be got from foods such as red grapes, onions, yellow and white ones, apples, broccoli and garlic.

- **Antioxidants.**

Antioxidants should be an integral part of everyone's diet. They help to protect the body from free radicals, which are responsible for triggering off inflammation. You will find a surprising number of foods that are rich in antioxidants including carrots and winter squash, because of the beta-carotene they contain, colorful bell peppers for their vitamin C, tomatoes for their lycopene and leafy greens, like kale, spinach, beet greens, Swiss chard and many others besides.

- **Omega-3 fatty acids.**

Omega-3 fatty acids are something that are sorely lacking in most of our diets. In fact, one of the biggest causes of inflammation is too much Omega-6 and not enough omega-3. Omega-3 fatty acids are full of benefits to anyone who has an inflammatory condition and the best ones are found cold seafood's like salmon, anchovies, sardines, herrings and also in walnuts, flaxseed and those all important dark leafy greens.

- **Oleic acid**.

Oleic acid is an omega-9 fatty acid, which is required for the omega-3 fatty acids to work properly. The best sources of this are macadamia nuts and almonds along with olive oil.

- **Curcumin.**

Perhaps better known to most of you as turmeric, this is an Indian spice, used to add flavor and color to curry and can be used in place of saffron to give a yellow color to rice as well. Turmeric is one of the single most powerful natural anti-inflammatory foods found today, just ahead of ginger and rosemary.

Chapter 5: Anti-inflammatory Foods

Almonds and Other Nuts

Nuts are well known for their anti-inflammatory nature and they are better than many anti-inflammatory foods. Almonds are almost on top of the list when it comes to anti-inflammatory foods. Walnuts are very helpful in rheumatoid arthritis; cashews are a very good choice as well. Main advantage of these nuts is that they are versatile and can be eaten in various ways. They are very delicious, sometimes can be served in place of snacks, and sometimes can be used as a flavoring agent in many dishes.

Carrots

Health professionals and enthusiasts always appreciate carrots and it is very easy to understand why. Carrots contain high levels of beta-carotene and Vitamin A. An easy way to eat more carrots is by drinking carrot juice. It is very difficult to eat lots of carrot to have all beneficial ingredients, so you can add some carrots in your smoothie to make it an anti-inflammatory smoothie.

Cinnamon

Cinnamon is a spice that can be obtained from the bark of many trees from Cinnamomum genus and is mainly used in many savory and sweet foods. Cinnamon is enriched with anti-oxidants that can help your body in several ways, but especially to reduce the inflammation in your body. In other words, by sprinkling a little amount of cinnamon on your foods, you are working to reduce the inflammation in your body.

Cucumber

Cucumber is a vegetable that has been gaining more focus from health experts. It is alkaline, ultra-hydrated, and rich in anti-oxidants and an anti-inflammatory food. The best thing about this green food is that it can be added in fresh salad that already has many anti-inflammatory foods. It can also be blended in green smoothies.

Apple Cider Vinegar

There are different uses of apple cider vinegar. It can be added into drinking water to purify it and it is often added in green smoothies and other detoxifying drinks because of its health benefits. The beauty of it is that you can add it to your beverages and foods to make them anti-inflammatory. The major benefit of apple cider vinegar is that it aids digestion and GIT, so you can see many benefits if you suffer from constipation, diarrhea or gastroenteritis. When you have a healthier digestive system, you can process the foods in a good way. Apple cider vinegar can also help in weight loss.

Apricots

You can add many fruits to your anti-inflammatory foods list and apricot is one of those foods. Inflammation is often related with phytochemicals and apricot can help in this regard by having a yellow crystalline pigment quercetin. Apricots can make your salad very delicious. Consider a salad made of almonds, spinach and apricots; this would be blend of anti-inflammatory foods.

Bell Peppers

Bell peppers possess anti-oxidant properties because of flavonoids. Bell peppers are valuable superfoods. These bright colored and beautiful peppers are enriched with many vital anti-oxidants that can help your body in different ways along with reducing inflammation. They can be used for different purposes like for weight loss, as they are a low calorie food. The anti-oxidants will help you combat free radical damage. Try to mix up different colors of these peppers so that you can have different flavonoids.

Fennel

The health benefits of fennel have been known to us for many years and now it is on the list of anti-inflammatory foods. It is on the list because of its phytonutrient and anti-oxidant values. Both these items help to ease the symptoms of inflammation and treat the causes of inflammation. If you are suffering from a chronic inflammation, you need to treat it in a comprehensive manner and you should focus on your diet. If you are not familiar with fennel, find some fennel recipes to make you use this amazing anti-inflammatory food.

Garlic

Garlic is a top anti-inflammatory food and all health experts believe that it contains anti-inflammatory properties. It is very common that garlic supplements are usually prescribed to battle chronic inflammation. The best way to use this natural anti-inflammatory food is to use in your cooking. If you notice an improvement in your inflammation symptoms by having more garlic in your diet, start eating in supplemental form as well. If you can eat them without caring about the taste, garlic supplements are the best way to eat garlic.

Green Tea and Other Types of Tea

There are plenty of health benefits associated with green

tea. The one obvious benefit if green tea is it can help you to fight against some types of cancer. It has a high anti-oxidant count that makes it the perfect addition to your daily routine. Along with green tea, some other herbal teas have anti-inflammatory properties. You need to carefully pick herbal teas that have flavonoids. The best thing about these herbal teas is that they are so easy to prepare and usually need hot water to prepare them.

Papaya

Papaya is not a popular fruit and not among the top selling fruits in the United States, but it is one of healthiest and nutritional fruit. It should be in your list if you are trying to follow an anti-inflammatory diet. It is worth noting that certain ingredients in papaya fruit are not commonly found in other fruits that make it a more important anti-inflammatory fruit. It is often used in fruit salad and tastes great when mixed with some other fruits. Once you get the skill on how to prepare this amazing fruit, you will love this fruit in its season.

Salmon

Salmon is the best food option among fish if you are trying to fight against inflammatory diseases or conditions. Salmon fish have a great amount of omega-3 and it has been verified several times that it has strong anti-inflammatory effects. Eating salmon and other types of fish that are high in omega 3 can help decrease the inflammation in a quick and great way. Interestingly, eating salmon fish can combat overeating omega-6 foods. Eating more omega-6 and less omega-3 food leads to inflammation.

Spinach

Spinach is among one of the vegetables that we should eat more and more as it packed with so many nutrients. It is packed with many valuable nutrients like proteins, fibers and phytonutrients. This is a vegetable we should eat so often. It is good if you eat this vegetable on a daily basis to help fight against cancer and heart diseases. It is among top anti-inflammatory foods and easily available throughout the year.

Cabbage

Try to have red cabbage when you can find it out there in the market to benefit from a vital ingredient it contains, the anthocyanin's. Red cabbage is believed to have a significant anti-inflammatory advantage over other types of cabbage. But you should not overlook other types as they all belong to cabbage family and can easily give an anti-inflammatory boost to your meals. The easiest way to have it in the soup form as it is easy to digest and chew in the soup form. It is easy and beneficial to make anti-inflammatory soup of cabbage and other green vegetables in bulk, store it and then drink it during your meals.

Blueberries and other berries

Blueberries and some other berries like blackberries and raspberries are full of anti-oxidants along with phytonutrients that make them anti-inflammatory fruits. That is why by having berries you can have double benefits of anti-oxidants that can help you protect from free radical damage, cancer, heart diseases and they can also help you to fight against inflammation that can make many of these diseases more severe. Moreover, all berries taste great and by eating them, you can start feeling awesome. You will often see them added in so many smoothies because of their cleansing and anti-oxidant properties.

Chapter 6: Why Processed Foods Are Bad For You

One thing you will notice about anti-inflammatory diets is that they advise you to totally avoid processed foods. That's because processed foods are linked to chronic inflammation and various health conditions that can be life limiting and even life threatening. But why are processed foods so bad for you, and why do they have no place in an anti-inflammatory diet?

Sugar content

Processed foods tend to be high in sugar content, and that's bad news for your health. Sugar has lots of calories, but no nutritional benefits to go with it. In other words, the calories you get from sugar are 'empty' calories. As if that wasn't bad enough, sugar can also adversely affect the metabolism, causing insulin resistance and energy spikes. Sugar is very quickly broken down by the body for energy, and this encourages the pancreas to produce more insulin. And when blood sugar levels are high, the body produces more free radicals. This in turn stimulates an immune system response, which triggers inflammation.

All of this is bad news for the body, because unused sugar also converts to triglycerides – fats that are instrumental in causing heart disease. Together with the inflammation that can damage the blood vessels around the heart, this can produce a serious situation health wise. The trouble is, the sugar content in processed food is not easily measured – a lot of it is hidden. It's there to extend the shelf life of the products and improve the taste, but all that comes at the expense of your health. And because of the high calorie count, sugar contributes to obesity, which also fuels internal inflammation.

The thing is, when you prepare your own meals, you have control over the amount of sugar that goes into them. That's not true when it comes to processed foods.

Low on nutrients, high on additives

During processing, many of the essential vitamins and nutrients that are vital to health – and also give foods their anti-inflammatory properties – are lost. Manufacturers get around this by fortifying the foods with synthetic vitamins, but the body is designed to take its nutrition from food sources. Synthetic vitamins are never going to pack the antioxidant punch of real vitamins obtained from real foods.

Plant and animal food sources also contain trace nutrients that simply can't be reproduced in a laboratory, so you really miss out on vitamins and minerals if you go for processed foods.

Processed foods also contain a number of chemicals and preservatives designed to prolong the shelf life of the products. The thing is, some of these chemicals don't even have to be named, as they are present in such small quantities. Do you really want to put extra chemicals in your body, dressed up as food?

The thing is with chemicals, you don't know how they're going to interact and react with the chemicals in your own body. It doesn't take much to disturb the body's delicate hormonal balance, and that can lead to all sorts of problems in later years. And if you don't have a name for the chemicals you are feeding into your body, you can't very well research them to see what possible problems they may cause.

Trans fats

Trans fats are perhaps the biggest threat to health, and you're only likely to find them in processed foods. Trans fatty acids – or trans fats as they are more commonly known – are created by a process of hydrogenation. Basically, hydrogen is added to liquid fats to make them more solid and stable. It's not a process you'd be likely to use at home, which is why you can be sure that nothing you produce in your kitchen will contain trans fats. That said, there are small amounts of naturally occurring trans fats in meat and some dairy products, but the harmful stuff comes from manufactured trans fats.

Ironically, the reasoning behind trans fats was to create a product that was healthier than butter, but in fact the reverse is true. Trans fats raise the amount of 'bad' LDL cholesterol in the blood. That's the kind that leads to clogged arteries and, subsequently, heart attacks and strokes. Trans fats also raise levels of blood triglycerides, which also contribute to heart problems and diabetes.

Around 40% of all processed foods contain some form of trans fats in varying quantities – even the so-called 'healthy' foods like granola bars and crackers. The only sure way to cut trans fats from your diet is to dispense with processed foods. By swapping trans fats for monounsaturated and polyunsaturated oils, you can reduce internal inflammation – since olive oil is one of the best things for that. Junking trans fats and limiting saturated fats can also cut your risk of developing diabetes by around 40%, and your chances of developing heart disease by more than 50%.

Low fiber content
Fiber is good for fighting internal inflammation and chronic health conditions such as heart disease and diabetes. However, during processing, a lot of the fiber is stripped from foods. Some processed foods may try to fool you by claiming to contain whole grains, but these

may not be in sufficient quantities to deliver the fiber hit you need for good health. Unless whole grains or oats are high on the list of ingredients, and a serving delivers a minimum of 3 grams of fiber, you're not getting enough. The problem is, most processed foods contain refined grains. That's not ideal, when studies show that getting enough fiber can reduce the risk of heart disease by between 20% and 30%. Low fiber intake is also linked to diabetes and some forms of cancer.

Salt content

Around 75% of the salt most people take in isn't added at the table or during cooking – it comes from the processed foods they eat. And the real problem is, you probably don't even know you're eating it, because it's there to preserve the food and enhance the flavor, rather than just as a seasoning. It's estimated that people who include a number of processed foods in their diets are consuming around twice as much sodium as they need for their health, so it's a major problem.

Salt occurs naturally in some of the natural foods everyone eats such as milk, celery, beets and even water. Some salt is necessary for health – it helps to regulate blood pressure and keep a healthy, natural fluid balance, by replacing fluid lost through sweating and other bodily functions.

However, if you take in more salt than your body needs, the body hangs onto fluids to dilute the sodium in the blood, and that can make the heart work harder, causing raised blood pressure. That's bad news for heart health. You can limit the amount of sodium in your diet by drastically reducing the level of processed foods in your diet. And if you really must have that pizza or ready-made pasta meal, check out the ingredients panel and go for the one with the least sodium content.

High fructose corn syrup (HFCS)

Some processed food manufacturers say that high fructose corn syrup is just a natural sweetener, and that it is healthier than sugar. However, the reverse is true. Neither sugar nor HFCS are healthy, because both contribute to obesity, and obesity is a key factor in internal inflammation and a number of chronic health conditions.

Scientifically, sucrose – or normal cane sugar – is composed of two bound molecules, fructose and glucose, which need to be broken down for digestive purposes before they are absorbed into the blood stream. HFCS is also comprised of glucose and fructose, but the molecules are not bound and are therefore more rapidly absorbed into the system. The fructose heads for the liver and triggers the release of unhealthy triglycerides and cholesterol, while the glucose causes insulin spikes. The net result is hormonal imbalances that make conditions like diabetes, weight gain, heart disease and cancer more likely.

The truth is, HFCS is usually found in poor quality, nutritionally deficient processed foods. That means that other unhealthy ingredients such as fat, salt and chemical additives are also likely to be present.

Processed foods have many unhealthy additives that are used to improve the flavor, appearance and shelf life of products. The result is that the real nutritional value and texture of the food is lost during the processing. If the additives in any way improved the taste experience of the health benefits, it would be different, but modern processed food is about as far removed from real food as is possible. It doesn't have to be time consuming or expensive to produce healthy, home cooked food, so junk the junk food and cook from scratch, using whole foods and natural ingredients.

Chapter 7: Cooking The Anti-Inflammatory Way

It's not just foods that have anti-inflammatory properties. The way you cook those foods can also impact on the effect they have on your body. Ideally, the least processing a food goes through, the more nutritional benefit you will gain from it, so where possible, eat foods raw, ready to eat and in season, because that will give your body maximum benefit. However, not all foods taste good raw, and indeed if you were to eat raw chicken, you're pretty much signing your own death warrant, so you need to be sensible about the whole thing.

Some foods, when cooked at high temperatures, can contribute to or exacerbate inflammation. That's because the cooking process produces advanced glycation end products – that's AGEs, which are also known as glycotoxins. The body produces AGEs during metabolism, and they are present in some food products derived from animals, but cooking certain foods at high temperatures produces new AGEs. High levels of these compounds in the body can trigger an inflammatory response, and have been linked to diabetes and heart disease.

Grilling, frying and microwaving foods – especially pork, beef, eggs and fish – increases the levels of AGEs. That doesn't mean you can never cook foods that way, just that you need to cut down a little. Steam, poach and slow cook, rather than searing and deep-frying. And counteract the effects of AGEs by including plenty of foods that are naturally low in the compound, such as fruits and vegetables. Ideally, these should be eaten raw or steamed, as that retains more of the vitamins and anti-oxidants. Anti-oxidants are known to counteract the effects of AGEs in the body.

Most people tend to sear and brown foods, particularly meats, before lowering the temperature to finish cooking, but by then the damage is done, because the browning is a sign that AGEs are present. Using a halogen oven does away with the need for searing – the food retains its moistness and flavor without the need for pre-browning. Also, cooking meat in a crock-pot or slow cooker will achieve the same end, so experiment with cooking methods.

Processed foods often contain AGEs, because they are cooked at very high temperatures, so that's yet another reason to avoid processed foods, if you didn't already have enough. Also, many of the packaging processes involve high temperatures. The fact is, the more processes a food goes through before it reaches your plate, the more chances there are of unhealthy compounds like AGEs being generated.

Poaching often gets a bad press, because most people's experience of poached food has been in hospitals, on special diets, when the poached food is bland looking and bland tasting. In reality, poached food – particularly chicken and fish – can be exceptionally tasty. It all depends on the poaching liquid. Use stock or wine flavored with herbs and spices rather than plain old boring water. Experiment, and find the best ways to poach your favorite foods. The poaching liquid can also be used as the base for a tasty sauce to accompany your food. If there is any fat in the food, allow the poaching liquid to cool, then skim off the fat before use to keep the fat content down in your diet.

Braising meats also cuts down on cooking temperatures and increases the flavor of the food. Another plus is that cuts for braising are often cheaper than other cuts of meat. So that's more proof that healthy food doesn't have to be expensive.

Another way to reduce AGEs in food is to cook them in vinegar or lemon juice – or another acidic medium. The same effect can be obtained by marinating beforehand. And in fact, marinating gives more flavor to food, which means you may not eat so much as normal, thus cutting down on both calories and AGEs.

Adding fat at the time of cooking, especially when cooking at high temperatures, also adds to AGE production. So, try not to add extra fat when cooking. And deep-frying really should be off the menu if you're concerned about internal inflammation.

Following an anti-inflammatory diet isn't just about eating the right foods – it's a whole approach to healthier eating. To follow a fully inflammatory lifestyle, you have to examine all aspects of your life, and make adjustments accordingly.

Chapter 8: Exercising To Beat Inflammation

As has just been mentioned, following an inflammatory diet isn't just about the foods you eat, it's about all aspects of your life and making healthy choices wherever you can. Exercise is a big part of the picture too. Chronic inflammation is a feature of life as you age, and exercise can help to mitigate this.

It's a fact that as we age, we are more prone to chronic inflammation. And while exercise can cause acute inflammation as a result of tissue damage, in the long term, exercise is beneficial in controlling chronic internal inflammation.

Studies have shown that exercising for around 20 minutes a day can reduce internal inflammation by around 12%, and that's just with moderate exercise. Also, your weight or fitness level doesn't really come into it. That would seem to be a powerful indication that exercise works when it comes to combating inflammation.

Immediately after exercise, the body produces and uses more anti-oxidants, which are known to help in the fight against inflammation. Also, exercise promotes the release of cytokines – protein molecules that can also help fight inflammation. Plus, exercise reduces stress, and stress is known to exacerbate chronic inflammation.

Exercise helps you to keep your weight in the healthy range, and it's well known that obesity is a big contributory factor in internal inflammation. So, what sort of exercise is good for combating inflammation? Well, basically anything that gets you moving and gets your heart working faster to pump the blood around your body. Aerobic exercise, combined with strength training, will work and tone your muscles, and boost the metabolism so you burn off any excess fat.

Another thing to consider is that fatty tissue encourages internal inflammation. If you embark on an exercise regime, the main aim will be to get rid of that fat and build muscle, and this is one of the best things you can do, either for yourself or someone you love.

Of course, exercise is only beneficial if you stick with it; so choose something you enjoy, that is easy to keep up and slots effortlessly into your lifestyle. Swimming, walking and cycling are good choices, since you can involve the rest of the family and don't need to invest in special equipment. Even dancing is great exercise – the important thing is consistency. Exercise needs to be planned and regular, with at least 20 minutes of moderate activity three to five times a week. To get the best results, you need to put in the effort every day. Let's take a look at the particular benefits of different exercises when it comes to combating inflammation.

Walking

Even 10 minutes of walking each day can reduce inflammation. Any sort of physical activity can do that, but walking is good, simply because it's an easy option. You don't need any specialist equipment, training, talent or aptitude to walk, and it's not a team sport, so you don't need to compete with anyone, and maybe suffer a nasty knock to your self-esteem. We learn to walk before we can talk – it's part of life.

You can walk alone, with friends, with children or with the dog, and if you walk with kids or dogs, you'll meet lots of new people who will want to admire and talk about your babies or your fur babies. That's great for stress relief, and stress is another cause of inflammation.

The thing with walking is you don't need to make a special effort to build it into your day. You can do it any time, because you don't need to travel to a class or set aside a specific time for walking. Therefore it feels like a natural part of your life, and that means you're more likely to stick with it. Don't worry if you can't walk too far or too fast to start with – you'll be surprised how quickly you'll build up strength, speed and stamina.

Another point to remember is that intensive exercise in bursts can actually add to the inflammation problem. It's preferable to exercise moderately and regularly, and that's where walking comes in. There are lots of ways you can build more walking into your day. Get off the bus a stop earlier, park the car further away, take the stairs instead of the elevator. If you don't have a dog, why not volunteer for dog walking duties at an animal shelter? Or set yourself up as a dog walker and earn some bucks as you fight inflammation. You just need the determination to do it, and you will manage to walk more.

If you walk for at least half an hour a day you'll boost your metabolism, which will in turn help you to lose any excess weight you may be carrying. Since obesity is a major cause of inflammation, trimming off those pounds will help enormously.

Swimming and water exercise

As has been mentioned before, exercise is something of a double-edged sword when it comes to fighting inflammation. Too much exertion is as bad as not enough, so you need to get the balance right. One way to do that is to make swimming your exercise of choice.

There are two real bonuses about exercising in water, whether you're swimming or doing aqua aerobics. The water supports your entire weight, whatever that may be. That means no undue stress is being placed on your joints, which is a common contributor to acute internal inflammation. Also, the water adds resistance, which means that exercises done in water are much more effective than those undertaken on land.

One excellent example of this is running or jogging. While it is excellent exercise, it's not suitable for everyone. Joggers are more prone to injury, which can exacerbate inflammation problems. And if you happen to live in a hot country, it can be difficult to maintain a regular running schedule. That means you are not getting maximum anti-inflammatory benefits from your exercise session, since sustained regular exercise combats inflammation better than anything. However, if you run in the pool or in the ocean, you're supporting your joints, keeping cool and getting some great inflammation-busting exercise.

Swimming is social exercise too – often, people go swimming with friends, partners or as a family. That means it's enjoyable, and you're more likely to keep it up. Remember in this case, the exercise isn't a quick fix to drop a dress size for your vacation; it's a lifetime project to combat unhealthy internal inflammation. You really need to keep it going, and swimming and aqua exercise are good ways to have fun while you shed those pounds.

Swimming and water exercise also have a calming effect, which helps to reduce stress levels. As stress is a significant contributor to inflammation, that's another good reason to get yourself wet as you get yourself fit.

Dancing

As well as being great fun, dancing is also effective as an aerobic exercise. It gets your blood pumping around the body, boosting the circulation and releasing 'feel good' hormones into the bloodstream to reduce stress levels. That means it's good for keeping your heart healthy, and reducing the risk factors for chronic

There are many different forms of dance, so there's sure to be one that is appropriate for your age, health condition and level of fitness. You can just head off to the local hop and make some moves on the floor, or you can take it a bit more seriously and sign up for dance classes. The point is, dancing gets you moving, and that's what you need to do to keep inflammation away from your door.

Dancing helps build strong bones and muscles, boosts co-ordination and helps build strength and stamina. And if you do it regularly, you will lose weight. It's all looking good for those who like to trip the light fantastic as a way of keeping inflammation under control. It's social exercise too – which means it doesn't actually feel like exercise at all. That means you are more likely to stick with it. That's an important consideration when planning for long term healthy living.

Cycling

Pretty much like dancing, cycling is sociable, as well as being a great form of aerobic exercise that can also help with weight loss. So once again, it ticks all the anti-inflammatory boxes. Perhaps the only thing that may put cycling out of consideration is that it requires a certain amount of skill, and of course you will need to buy, borrow or lease a bike for your cycling sessions, so there's an element of expense involved as well.

Cycling is low impact exercise, so there's less chance of injury or causing muscle damage that can contribute to inflammation. It's possible to burn around 650 calories an hour when you undertake a strenuous bike ride, so it also kick starts the metabolism. If you need to lose some weight, cycling will help you to do it as well as building strength and stamina and toning your muscles. All these things can help control inflammation in the body.

You can achieve similar benefits by using a stationary exercise cycle, if you're a bit wary about cycling on the open road. However, you may miss out on the mood lifting element, since stationary cycling can be a bit boring. If that's the case, why not try a spinning class?

Spinning is the latest craze to hit the fitness world, and it has a lot going for it as an exercise form. It's conducted on specially adapted stationary bikes to music, and it's an intense yet low impact workout that exercises every part of the body, burning up around 600 calories a session, so it really will get you fit and tone your body.

Spinning instructors are specially trained to motivate their clients, so they get the maximum benefit from the workout, and as well as they physical benefits, there are a number or psychological pluses to spinning. It helps to build a positive mental attitude, which can be a great help when dealing with a chronic disease of the autoimmune system on a daily basis. Like other exercises, spinning releases endorphins into the body, which promote a 'feel good' mood which can last for a number of hours after the session has ended.

Moderate, regular exercise encourages the body to produce more antioxidants, as well as reducing levels of C-Reactive Protein (CRP), the substance responsible for inflammation. This double hit reduces the risks of developing serious conditions such as coronary heart disease, as well as helping to control pain levels naturally for people with autoimmune diseases.

It makes sense to fit at least 30 minutes of regular exercise into each day if you possibly can. However, any exercise is better than none, so ask your doctor's advice on this, and stop exercising when you feel pain, as this could be a sign that your inflammation levels are increasing. Be careful out there, and exercise wisely, but not too well. Have respect for your body and your immune system, and don't push it too hard.

Chapter 9: Natural Supplements Which Help Combat Inflammation

As has been mentioned before, many foods can help combat inflammation, thereby providing some natural pain relief for people suffering from autoimmune diseases. In addition, there are a number of natural supplements that can also help.

More people are looking for natural ingredients to fight inflammation, as many over the counter and prescription remedies can cause internal bleeding and stomach ulcers. The main problem with this is that often symptoms don't present until the condition is well advanced, by which time the patient may be seriously ill. Also, some anti-inflammatory medications can cause a decrease in the infection-fighting white blood cells. There are no nasty side effects with the supplements detailed below, and while they may not work for everyone, they certainly won't do any harm, so it's worth trying one or more of them, to see if they can afford you some natural pain relief.

Always consult your doctor before taking anything, no matter how safe and natural it seems, as there may be contraindications in your particular case. And don't expect supplements to work as quickly as NSAIDs. It takes a few weeks of regular use before you see the benefits, but you will. With all that in mind, these are some natural supplements you may wish to consider to help combat inflammation and relieve pain.

Turmeric

Turmeric has been used for centuries as a natural anti-inflammatory in Chinese and Indian medicine, and today it is enjoying a renaissance. The active ingredient is curcumin, and research indicates that this is as strong as hydrocortisone – which is a steroid – and other anti-inflammatory medications.

In the case of Rheumatoid Arthritis, (RA) turmeric is as effective at treating the condition as phenylbutazone, a non-steroidal anti-inflammatory drug (NSAID) that is no longer approved for human use in some countries. And it doesn't need to be taken in large doses either to achieve results. Circumin is a powerful antioxidant, which means it mops up the free radicals that are responsible for joint inflammation and damage.

People who regularly use the spice report an improvement in the severity and duration of early morning joint stiffness, as well as finding they have increased mobility, since they are experiencing less pain. This of course has a knock on effect – the more you exercise, the more supple and flexible your joints become, and the more you are able to exercise.

Curcumin also plays a major part in lowering cholesterol, which reduces the risk of coronary heart disease. This is a real concern in autoimmune diseases, as is the risk of developing cancer. When the body has a compromised immune system, it becomes more difficult, and even impossible, to fight off threats to the health. This mighty spice can achieve that.

If you're not keen on curries, there are still ways to incorporate turmeric into your diet. Add to mayonnaise-based salads and salad dressings for enhanced flavor and color, or use when steaming vegetables. Cauliflower, green beans and lentils all pair well with turmeric, and it's delicious in a rice and raisin salad. Turmeric is also used in mustard, so use it liberally as a condiment, and add turmeric to soups, stews and casseroles. Try and enjoy some turmeric every day, in one way or another.

It's also possible to make turmeric tea. For basic turmeric tea, just simmer a teaspoon of turmeric in boiling water for 10 minutes, strain and add lemon for flavor. It can also be brewed with cinnamon or ginger, which also have anti-inflammatory properties, and it can be sweetened with a little honey if the flavor is too bitter for your liking. Choose good quality ground turmeric for this, or for even better results, buy a fresh root and grate it yourself. This will give a superior flavor and enhanced health benefits.

Curcumin is also available as a supplement in capsule form, but it's better to get it straight from the food source, as the body is better able to process it in that way. Another consideration is that with capsules, it's possible to overdose on circumin – this is unlikely to happen when using it in food or tea. 250 – 500 milligrams is considered a safe dose – any more could lead to stomach problems and blood clotting issues in some individuals. Your doctor can advise on the best way to use turmeric.

The really good thing about turmeric is that it usually agrees with everyone. Most people can tolerate it, and the flavor is not too strong for most palates. If you're still skeptical about the health benefits of turmeric, you should know that on the Japanese island of Okinawa, where turmeric tea is enjoyed regularly, the average life expectancy is around 82 years!

Aloe vera

Most people are aware of the extraordinary healing powers of aloe vera for skin conditions and sunburn, and it is a common ingredient in skin care products – particularly anti-aging creams. However, it is also a powerful anti-inflammatory agent. The active ingredients are the plant sterols Campesterol and Bradykinin. Campesterol lowers cholesterol and reduces inflammation by generating new body cells to repair damage to cartilage and joints. It's therefore a very powerful supplement for autoimmune conditions such as Rheumatoid arthritis (RA) and Lupus.

Bradykinin helps boost the circulation by improving blood flow and allowing oxygenated blood to circulate through the body to increase mobility and assist the healing process. It's also a natural analgesic, so it helps with pain relief. Both compounds work well in tandem with other supplements and medication, and are easily tolerated by most people, with no significant side effects or contraindications. This is important, since some sterols can work against each other and inhibit the effectiveness of one or more supplements.

While aloe can be used as a topical treatment, the best way to treat inflammation with aloe is to take it internally, either as a gel or juice, or in crystallized form as a healthy snack. Aloe also contains salicylic acid, which is found in aspirin. However, taking the substance via aloe will not result in the stomach problems commonly associated with regular consumption of aspirin.

In fact, it may be more effective to combine both methods. You can buy aloe vera juice, or make your own. If you buy juice, make sure it has a high proportion of aloe included. It's fairly simple to make your own juice, as long as you have a plant that is truly therapeutic. The most effective one is called 'True Aloe,' and its botanical name is Aloe Barbadensis Miller. Use the more mature leaves, those nearest the ground, where the tips of the leaves are drying out, as the gel in these is more powerful and therefore more effective in treating inflammation.

A whole aloe vera leaf will contain enough gel to make 2 – 3 liters of juice, but if you want to make a single liter, you need a piece of leaf about 4 – 6 inches in length. Don't cut the leaf until you're ready to make the gel, since storing it will cause it to lose its powerful healing properties.

Carefully separate the inner gel from the leaf, using a small spoon, or removing the outer covering of the leaf so you can scoop out the inner gel. Be careful not to take up the yellow substance called aloin, as this can be irritating to the stomach. Simply whizz the gel to a smooth paste in a blender, then add 2 tablespoons (30 mls, or 1 ounce) to 250 mls of water.

This is the minimum daily dose for therapeutic benefits. The safe recommended dose is between 60 and 120 mls (2 – 4 ounces). Your doctor will advise you on the most appropriate dose in your case. If you prefer, you can mix the gel with fruit juice or almond milk, or add some honey to sweeten it. It's very versatile, and you should find lots of ways to use your aloe gel on the internet. Remember you can also use it as a topical treatment for skin irritations, sunburn and healing wounds.

Store the remaining aloe gel in the fridge, but use within a few days to ensure you receive all the healing properties. It's best to drink your aloe vera juice first thing in the morning, and at least 20 minutes before food, so that the juice can start to work its magic in your body before the body has to get busy on the digestive process.

Cod liver oil

For generations, cod liver oil has been recognized as having major health benefits, and many a child has been forced to endure the daily dose over the years because it would 'Help them to grow big and strong.' However, in recent years, this natural supplement has been sidelined by other, more glamorous-sounding remedies.

As far as fighting inflammation is concerned, cod liver oil, and other fish oils, can bring about a big improvement in the body when taken regularly. The good news is, these days it's possible to get your fish oil in capsule form, which avoids the unpleasant sensation of tasting fish oil every time you burp or cough for hours on end.

Cod liver oil is high in healthy Omega-3 fatty acids, notably docosohexenoic acid (DHA) and EPA, or eicospantenoic acid. That's a bit of a mouthful, but these important Omega-3s do a whole lot of good stuff in the body. For many years now, researchers and doctors have recognized the link between internal inflammation and coronary heart disease, and Omega-3s can address both those conditions. That's good news for people living with chronic autoimmune system conditions, since they are also at increased risk of heart disease.

DHA and EPA do a sterling job inside the body. They help to thin the blood, reducing the risk of stroke, as well as lowering 'bad' LDL cholesterol while raising levels of 'good' HDL cholesterol, and regulating blood pressure. All this serves to boost the circulation, so the joints and muscles get lots of healthy, oxygenated blood. Within three months of supplementing with cod liver oil or other, high quality fish oils, many people with joint problems report significant reduction in pain levels, along with increased mobility, so it's definitely worth a go.

Ensure you use a high quality cod liver oil or fish oil, and ask your doctor about the recommended dosage. Also, try to eat at least two servings of oily fish such as salmon, tuna or sardines each week, in order to obtain more Omega-3s.

Green tea

There are three main types of tea – black tea, green tea and oolong. It's a drink that has been enjoyed for centuries, and after water, it's the most consumed beverage in the world. More people enjoy a morning cup of tea than a morning coffee, despite the international stranglehold of Starbucks!

Of the three types of tea, green tea goes through less processing, and this means levels of plant polyphenols – which are powerful antioxidants – are much higher in green tea. The leaves are not fermented, as they are in black tea. Green tea also helps to boost the metabolism, so it can be useful for weight loss. Losing excess weight is a great benefit for people with chronic autoimmune disease, because not only does it relieve the stress on damaged joints and muscles, but being overweight is linked to increased levels of internal inflammation.

Another useful benefit of drinking green tea is that it helps the body to fight off infections. That's important if you have a compromised immune system – you need all the help you can get in repelling invaders. Green tea is also believed to prevent and inhibit damage to cartilage and soft tissues, making it a healthy and flavorful drink for people with any form of arthritis or autoimmune disease. Two to three cups a day will help reduce inflammation and mop up the free radicals that can cause some forms of cancer and heart disease.

Vitamin C

The main value of vitamin C as a supplement is that it helps boost the immune system and fight infection. That's important when the immune system is compromised due to an autoimmune disease, or the drugs necessary for treatment. Anti-inflammatory drugs can also deplete your levels of vitamin C, and since the body cannot store this vitamin, you may benefit from taking a supplement, as well as including plenty of fruits in your diet to get the required amount of vitamin C.

Vitamin C helps renew the body's cells, and assists the body in making collagen, which is essential for building healthy cartilage, ligaments and tendons to protect and strengthen the joints. Smoking depletes levels of vitamin C so if you smoke, you should quit as soon as possible.

The most pleasant way to take it is as a soluble, effervescent dose in water. It makes a pleasant drink, and a daily dose of 1 gram will maintain healthy levels of vitamin C in the body to help fight infection and mop up the free radicals that cause inflammation and chronic disease. Do not take more than 1 gram of vitamin C as a supplement unless your doctor advises it, and overdosing on vitamin C can damage the kidneys and cause a number of side effects including diarrhea, headaches and nausea. Nobody should take more than 2 grams of vitamin C a day.

While all of these supplements can help fight inflammation and therefore alleviate the problems of autoimmune diseases, there may be clinical reasons why one or more of them is not suitable for you. Check with your doctor, and ensure you are eating a healthy, balanced diet, because supplements are meant to supplement the diet, not replace healthy, nutritious foods. Also, the body is designed to extract nutrients from food sources rather than synthetic forms, so be sure you understand the effects supplements are likely to have on your body and your condition before taking anything.

The great thing about treating autoimmune conditions with anti-inflammatory foods and supplements is that there are few or no side effects, and your general health will benefit as well as your specific condition. Read up on the benefits of anti-inflammatory foods and natural supplements and introduce as many as you can into your life. Together with the right amount of appropriate exercise, these natural solutions can bring about a major improvement in your quality of life, and the really good news is, you are taking back control of your body.

Conclusion

Well, after reading this book, you are well aware of inflammation, why it is helpful and harmful at the same time, how to decrease it and how and what natural foods can help you fight against auto-inflammatory diseases and inflammation. Inflammation is the response of the immune system to certain infections, injuries and to environmental triggers. Basically, inflammation is not bad itself and it can be helpful for the body. Simply, without inflammation, you cannot heal. But when left untreated and unmonitored, it can lead into chronic inflammation and can cause some serious health problems and diseases like cancer, rheumatoid arthritis and heart diseases. This is why chronic inflammation is dangerous and should be treated with great care and attention.

There are so many medications in the market today to treat inflammation and inflammatory diseases like steroids and NSAIDS. But the problem is that you cannot use these drugs for a long time because of associated side effects and their damaging effects on the immune system. So what should be done to battle inflammation? Nature is so wise as Nature has provided us with so many natural anti-inflammatory foods that can be used not only to fight against inflammation, but, by regularly eating them, we can stop inflammation, inflammatory diseases and conditions and keep ourselves healthy and strong.

You May Enjoy My Other Books

Below you'll find some of my other popular books on Amazon. You can also visit my author page.

hyperurl.co/MarySolomon

TIBETAN SECRETS: Five Steps To Unlimited Energy And Restored Health

smarturl.it/5rites

HEALING: Heal Your Body Heal Your Life

smarturl.it/healingaa

AUTOIMMUNE DISEASE ANTI-INFLAMMATORY DIET

smarturl.it/autoa

CRYSTAL HEALING ENERGY

smarturl.it/crystala

CHAKRA HEALING EXPOSED

smarturl.it/chakraaa

MEDICAL MARIJUANA and Pain Free Living

smarturl.it/mja

Happiness and LAW OF ATTRACTION

smarturl.it/loaa

www.ingramcontent.com/pod-product-compliance
Lightning Source LLC
Chambersburg PA
CBHW070913180526
45168CB00005B/2007